A Serendipitous Journey to the Magic Bullet

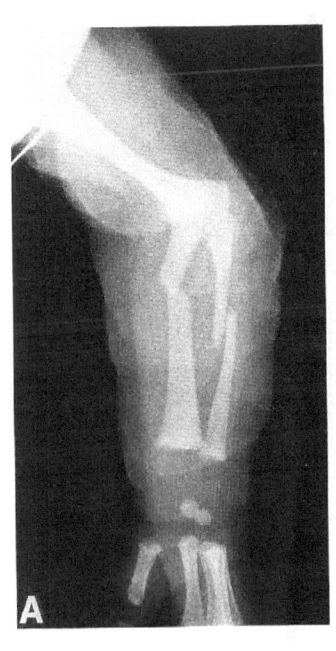
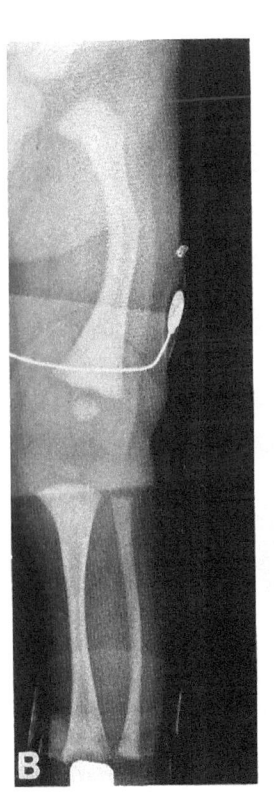

By: Marcie Brock

A Serendipitous Journey
to the Magic Bullet

By: Marcie Brock

www.marciebrockbooks.com

Other Books by Marcie Brock

Through Jake's Eyes: A Grandmother's Creation of Love
(2014)

Published by
Sue Breeding
Creating-Design
P.O. Box 1785
Columbus, IN 47202

Reason Behind the Book

I received an email from my orthopedic surgeon asking if I would talk to his patient about a rare, elbow operation that was performed on me. The patient, whose arms were fused at birth like mine, was unsure whether to have a surgery that would mobilize the arms, because of the outcome. Upon my agreement, I received the patient's email and wrote a lengthly letter about how I kept my arms mobile after the procedure. It's no secret that orthopedic surgeries are hard to recover from, but dedication and determination results in a successful outcome. The patient ended up moving forward with the operation after my letter of encouragement. My goal is to help others with a similar medical situation.

Imagine living with cardboard wrapped around your elbows and not being able to move them for years. That's the way I lived my life for sixteen years. Living with Antely-Bixler Syndrome resulted in fused elbows.

My right elbow broke while my mother was giving birth to me.

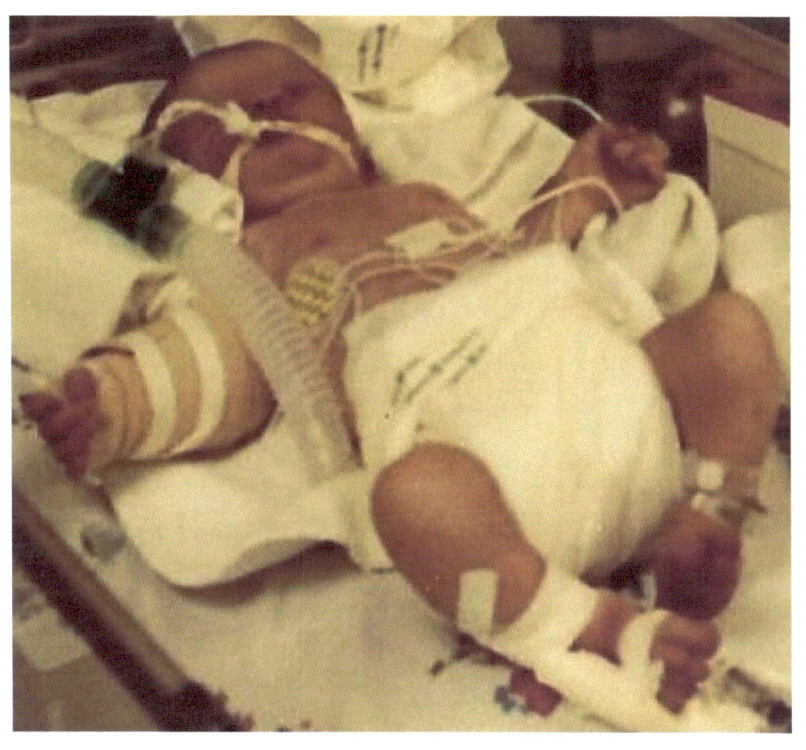

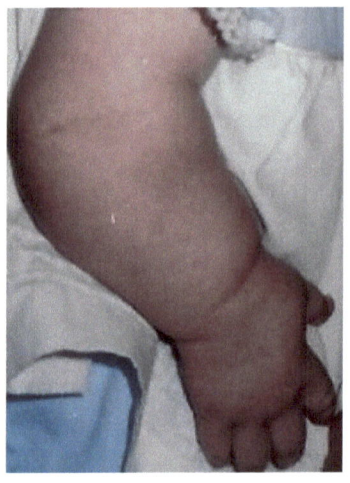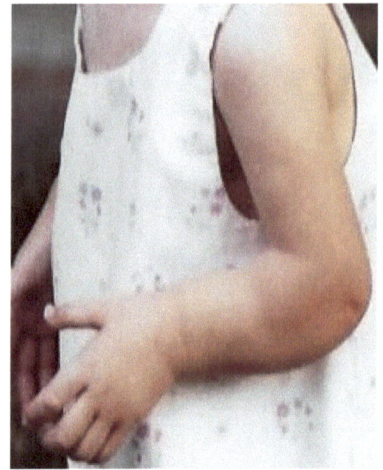

Doctors set my right elbow at a ninety-degree angle when they put on the cast. My left elbow, however, was fixed at eighty degrees.

Unfortunately, science wasn't perfected at that time to help patients with these unique elbows. Therefore, doctors told my distraught parents that nothing could be done. One doctor even told my parents that if I could eat with one hand and wipe with the other, nothing needed done. However, neither he nor most other orthopedic doctors could ever understand the difficulty of my life or other patients' lives.

All children want to become independent from their family when they get older, but some children achieve it easier than others. Daily routines such as bathing, eating, putting on clothes, necklaces, earrings, or make-up, along with washing and styling hair are some main essentials to that freedom. Kids who find these necessities an easy accomplishment are unaware that there are other people who find it a challenge.

These everyday adventures were challenging for me. I had to use a sponge with a handle to bathe myself. My mother would have to wash my hair in the sink and style it the way I wanted. I didn't mind it as a kid but as I entered my teenage years, it was increasingly irritating because I wanted to be like my friends and do it myself. It was a chore to cut up food and eat since my immobile elbows caused me to hold silverware a certain way. My arm immobility made it difficult to dress myself because some clothing styles needed my arms to bend a certain way. Imagine the awkwardness of having to ask for help getting dressed. Buttoning-up shirts was a problem because my arms wouldn't reach some of the buttons. Putting on necklaces, earrings, or makeup was difficult and became self-esteem issues. Scratching my neck or back was impossible. My fused elbows wouldn't let me smack mosquitoes or bugs when they bit me. As I grew older and wanted my own independence, the frustration of daily routines continued to increase. My only hope was a cure.

Never giving up hope was the key to finding the cure but not without heartache first. When I was ten years old, my growth and development doctor, Dr. Marilyn Bull, suggested I see Dr. Alexander Mih, a pediatric orthopedic surgeon at Riley Hospital for Children in Indianapolis. My mother scheduled an appointment in hopes of hearing answers we desperately needed. However, I had already learned by the age of ten that every high point starts with a low point. Upon observing the ordered X-Ray, I heard a familiar, depressing statement, "There is nothing the medical field can do for you at the present time, Marcie. Research is being done on this but there's no 'magic bullet.'" The letdown gave me the urge to shake him and say; "Do you have any idea how difficult it is to live with fused elbows?" However, I knew, with the current research, he wasn't comfortable doing surgery at that time.

Still, the only determination I needed in order to continue searching was the tears in my mother's eyes, the disappointment in my father's face, and my constant everyday struggles. I knew it was going to take a scientific miracle to solve my problem. Persistence and patience eventually paid off. My Aunt Mary Ellen knew we were looking for answers and told us she worked with an anesthesiologist who knew an orthopedic doctor in Canada. My mother called the Canadian doctor, and he thought he could help me since my arm muscles allowed me to write. The doctor was willing to do the needed elbow surgery for free, but finding a hospital was an issue. Unfortunately, we couldn't further pursue with the Canadian doctor, at that time, because I was set to have back surgery to correct scoliosis and kyphosis. However, sometimes you have to thank God for unanswered prayers.

Sometimes a miraculous solution comes by serendipity. Following my back surgery, I was required to have extensive physical therapy to regain strength. One therapy session was God's answer to my eventual freedom. While having therapy, my mother was flipping through a Family Circle magazine when she came across an article about a doctor who helped save a shoulder of a Columbine shooting victim. My mother wondered if this doctor could help me, so following therapy, we rushed to a computer and typed in the doctor's name in order find an email address. We sent an email to the doctor about my problem and received a reply from his secretary. She asked if we had seen the "60-Minutes" television special, during that week, on new medical advancements that enable doctors to help patients with limited mobility in their extremities such as hands, elbows, and knees. We told her "No" but read an article about the doctor in the <u>Family Circle</u> magazine. The secretary said hundreds of letters were received following the special; and a committee pulled out ones they thought they could help. My mother's letter about my problem was one, which they chose. She also said the committee was going to review my case to see which doctor would best fit my needs and get back with us within a couple of days. True to her word, she called back and told us they thought a doctor in Mayo Clinic in Rochester, Minnesota, by the name of Dr. James Morey, could help me move one step closer towards independence. No further time was wasted and an appointment was made for late December 2010, despite my dad reminding us the possible ramifications of traveling in Minnesota's treacherous winters. I felt my time was now and couldn't turn down this opportunity.

Mother Nature made sure I was going to have to earn my liberty as she released her ferocious wrath on our way up to Mayo Clinic. Radio stations kept telling people to stay off the highways as we crept through Minnesota's snowy roads. We saw cars, trucks, and semis flipped over on the side of the road and faced a wind chill factor of minus 30 degrees Fahrenheit. I remember my brother, who was sitting in the front seat with Dad, telling us how nuts we were and that if he did anything like this, Dad would have a fit, which was true. Dad could only see a foot in front of him but after my family and I prayed a lot, we finally made it to our hotel in Rochester, Minnesota. My adventurous road to freedom was just beginning.

A mid-December morning was the day I had been waiting for all sixteen years of my life. I woke up excited about the opportunity of my forthcoming independence even though a little negativity was in the back of my mind because of past disappointments. "What if this is a wasted trip and he is going to tell me what all the other past doctors told me, 'Nothing can be done at this time as there is no magic bullet?" Still, I had learned to keep stepping forward and never look back.

Walking through Mayo Clinic's doors was like walking through the gates of Heaven I was given a new outlook on life. Dr. Morey and I agreed to focus on the right arm first since it is my dominant arm. I underwent a series of tests including an X-Ray and a nerve test, where a technician stuck a needle into different spots on my arm to see if the nerves could send messages to my arm to move. Once undergoing a series of tests, Dr. Morey reviewed the tests and examined my right elbow. Upon examination, he uttered the most beautiful words a doctor could say to a patient who was considering undergoing a potential, life-changing operation, "When are you looking to have this done?" I looked over at my relieved mother and saw a gleam in her eyes when she asked, "You think you can really help her?" Dr. Morey, with a smile on his face, said he saw no reason not to do the surgery from what he saw of my apparent determination and my functional arm muscles. After he exited the room, I noticed Mom's happy tears in her eyes. I looked at the heavens smiling, winking, and mouthing, "Thank you." I realized the opportunity had been given when the secretary scheduled the surgery for mid June 2001. Preparation was underway for the life-changing procedure.

I was willing to do anything and everything to get functional elbows. Dr. Morey stated the best result would be gained if I built more muscles. My parents bought me a gym membership so I could lift weights and use their exercise machines. I obviously couldn't use the machines properly because of my immovable elbows; but that didn't stop me. My willpower continued as I also lifted weights at home. I hadn't come this far to let this opportunity slip away. Each passing day meant one step closer to independence. Excitement grew at the thought of doing things I couldn't do before because of my non-functioning elbows. My life was forever changing, as

I was about to feel reborn. I hardly slept the night before the surgery as I lay in bed thinking about the future. It was time to face a grueling war!

Not knowing the end result would be both exciting and scary. I was overwhelmed with mixed emotions on the morning of a potentially life-changing surgery. Nervousness started kicking in. My outer self was excited for my future, but my inner self prepared for the worse. The two main things I worried about were anesthesia problems and whether I had prepared enough for this big day. There was no room for butterflies in my stomach because I had come too far to back down.

While being prepped for surgery, the anesthesiologist told me an anesthesia block would be inserted around my armpit to numb the elbow following surgery. That didn't faze me. I was ready to end the suspense of what would happen in the aftermath of the surgery as I finally would see my elbow move and how excited I would feel when Dr. Morey informed me of the success of the life-changing operation. Prior to entering the operating room, I kissed my right arm goodbye and said; "Time to breathe."

For me, the unknown end result of this surgery was nerve-wracking. As the sedation wore off, my ears heard some wonderful 'music' from Dr. Morey;

"Good news! The surgery was a success. Your arm is moving." As I slowly widened my eyes, I looked down at my right arm and noticed it was straight for the first time in 16 years. I breathed a sigh of relief.

Once stable, I was wheeled to my room knowing I had a long road ahead. Therapists soon realized they would be dealing with a gritty patient. There was no time for laziness as therapists stressed the importance of keeping the arm mobile. They immediately demonstrated the bedside Continuous Passive Motion (CPM) machine by placing my arm in a splint-like contraption and moving my arm to flexion and extension twenty-four hours a day. I was told to be on it until physical therapy time.

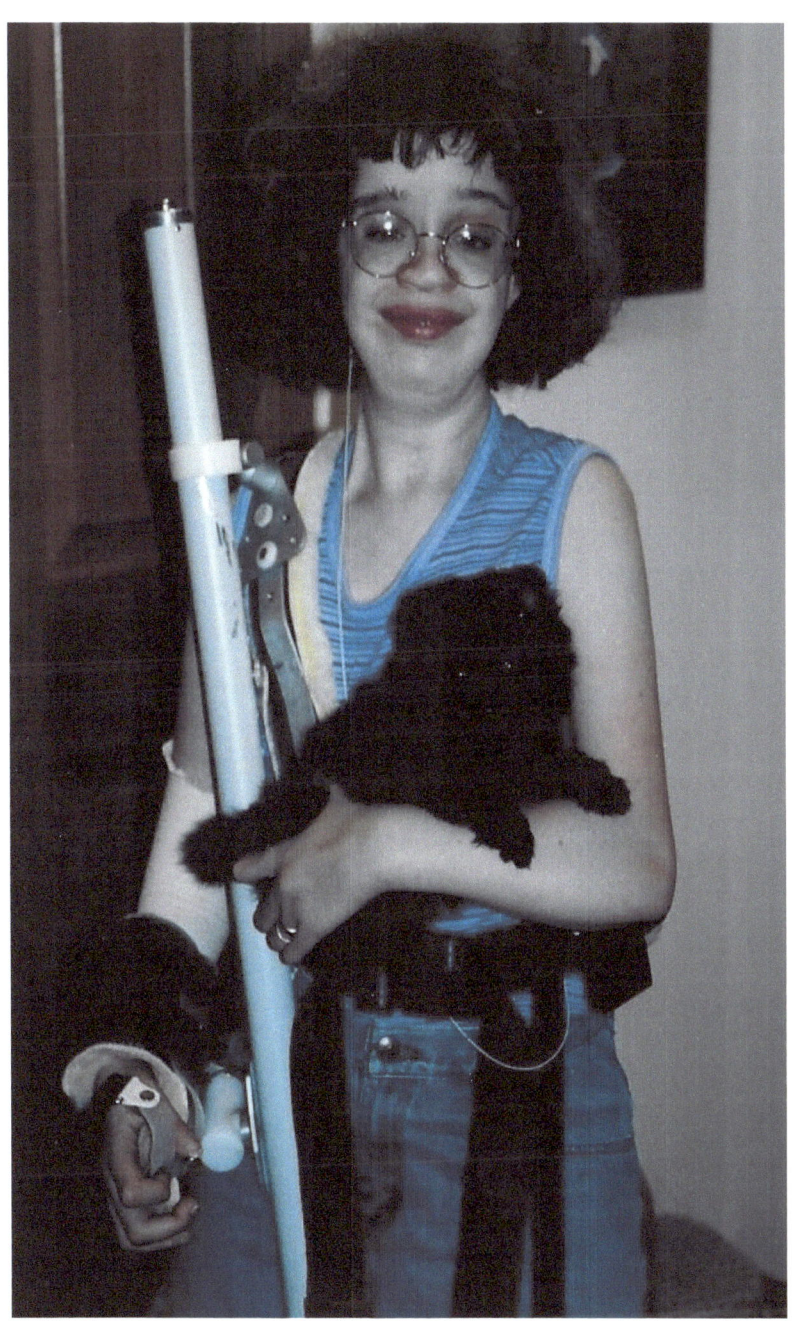

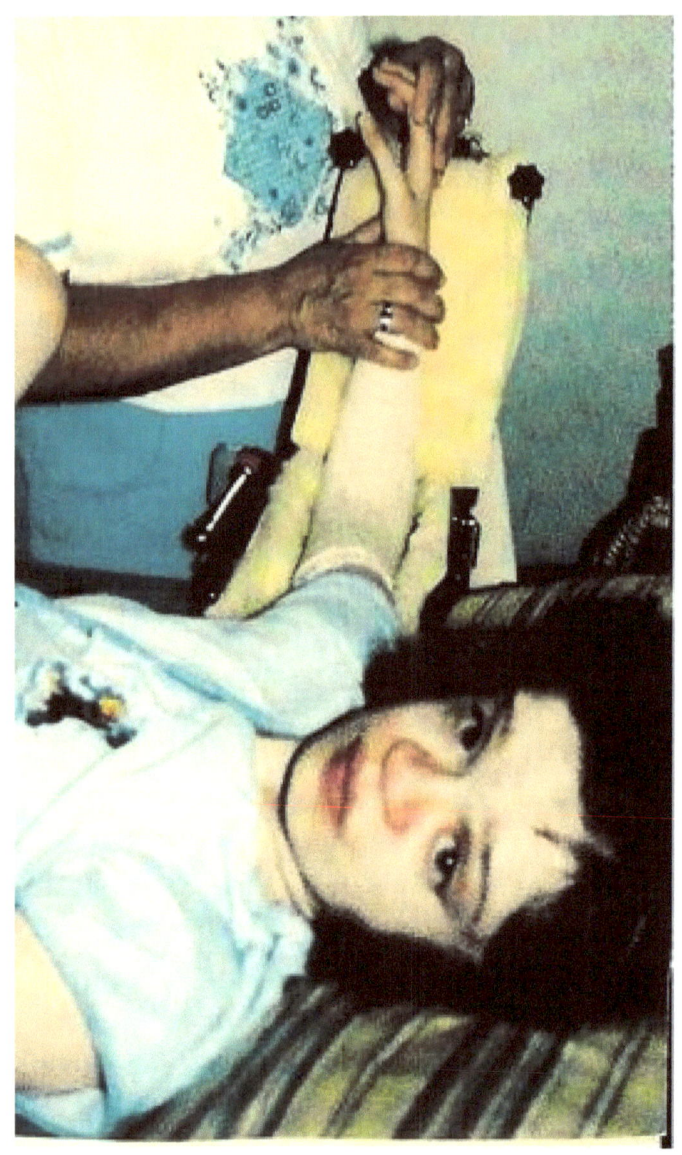

If I wanted to sit-up out of the bed then I was to be on a portable CPM machine, which was a three-foot-long, battery-operated pole with a cuff strapped to my arm. I felt right on schedule with my recovery, but every road to success seems to have speed bumps along the way.

Nurses got a run for their money because it's not easy to care for a patient with an unknown surgery result. I was unaware of the amount of pain I'd have after surgery, so imagine my shock when the pain seemed unmanageable. I received routine pain medication where nurses stuck a needle in the under part of my arm to numb my arm and block the pain. However, something went terribly wrong the second day after surgery. While I don't remember the incident, my mother stated I was complaining of mouth numbness; the next thing I knew I heard people calling my name to wake up. Apparently, an unknown entity tested my toughness as I had a seizure when the needle got too close to a vein, causing the medication to go to the bloodstream. I was momentarily knocked down but quickly got back up. Four days later, Dr. James Morey informed me he felt confident enough to release me from the hospital but not without discharge instructions.

Prior to my release, nurses gave me instructions to follow at home along with medication scripts to fill and pill to take for pain. Afterwards, I was instructed by therapists to wear the portable CPM machine out of the hospital and during the ten-hour ride home. It proved to be challenging because the machine and I barely fit in the backseat of the Dodge Neon. While at home, I had to use the bedside CPM machine that plugged into the wall. If I wanted to get out of the house, I had to use the portable one to keep my arm mobile. When not on the machine, I wore a variety of splints. I wore the custom, molded flexion and extension splints for a half hour at a time in between the CPM machine.

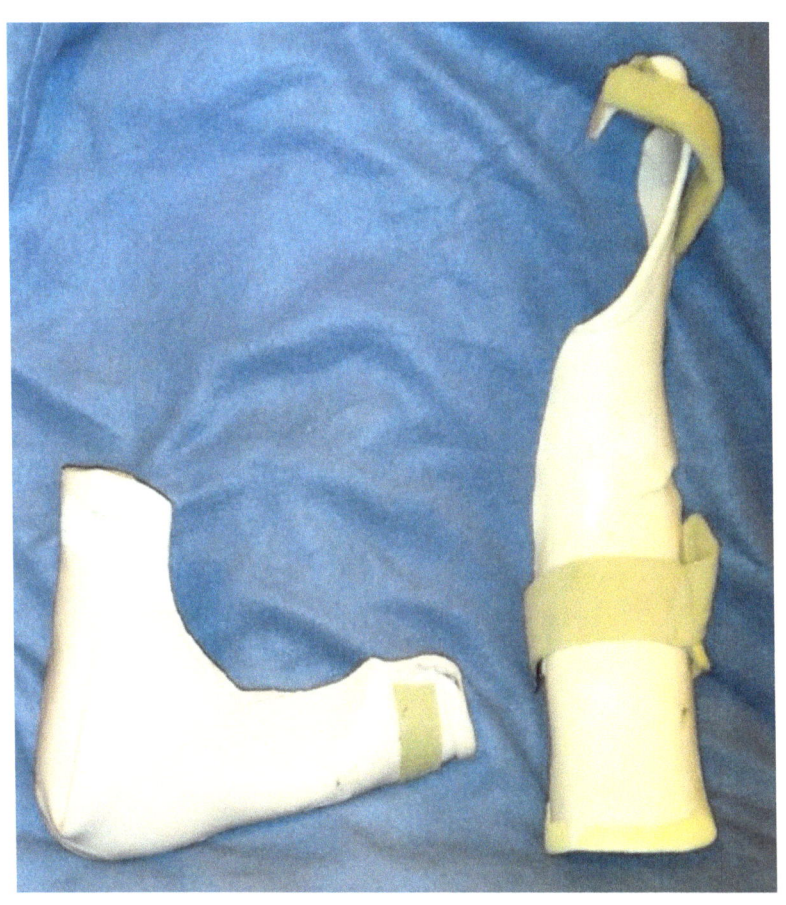

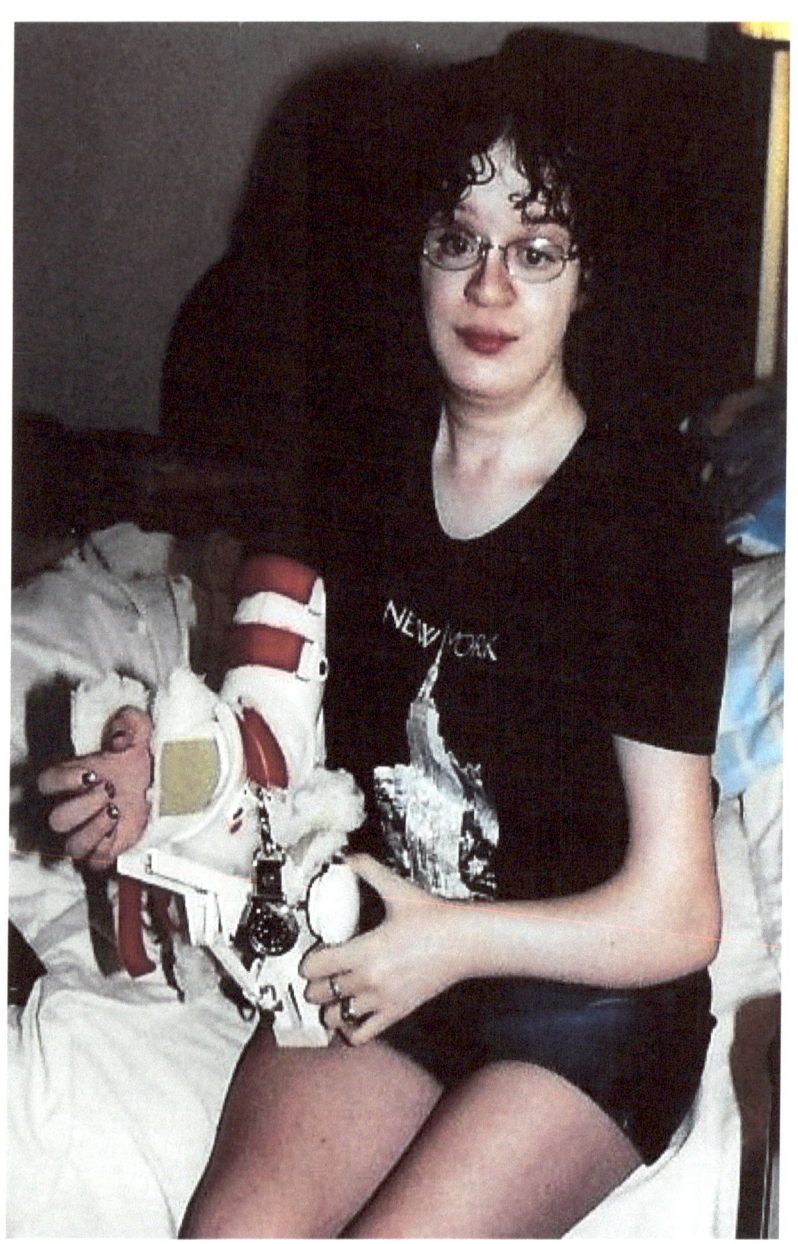

Along with the custom splints and CPM machine, I also cranked my arm to flexion and extension every 30 minutes respectively for one hour in the Joint Active Splint (JAS). Additionally, I attended physical therapy three times a week along with doing home therapy. Resting my arm from the machine, splints, or therapy wasn't an option as it meant a victory for scar tissue.

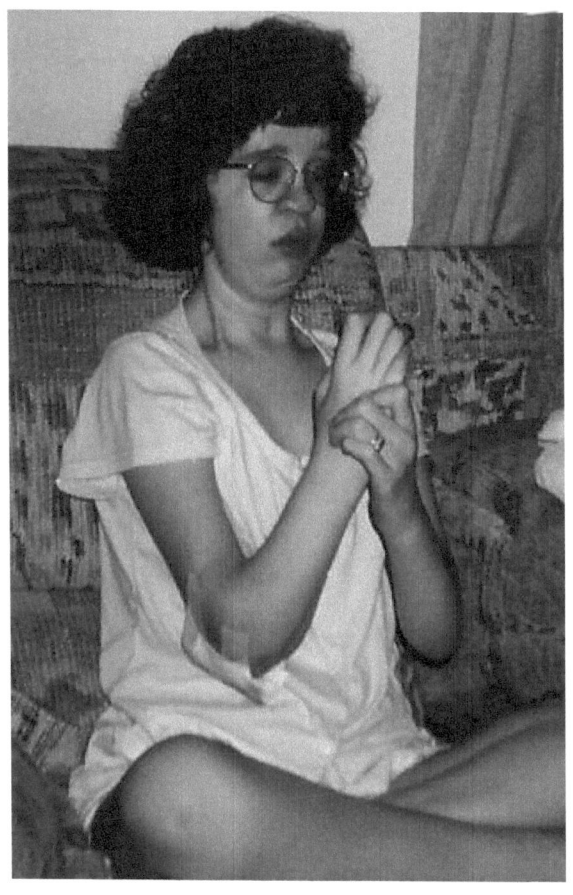

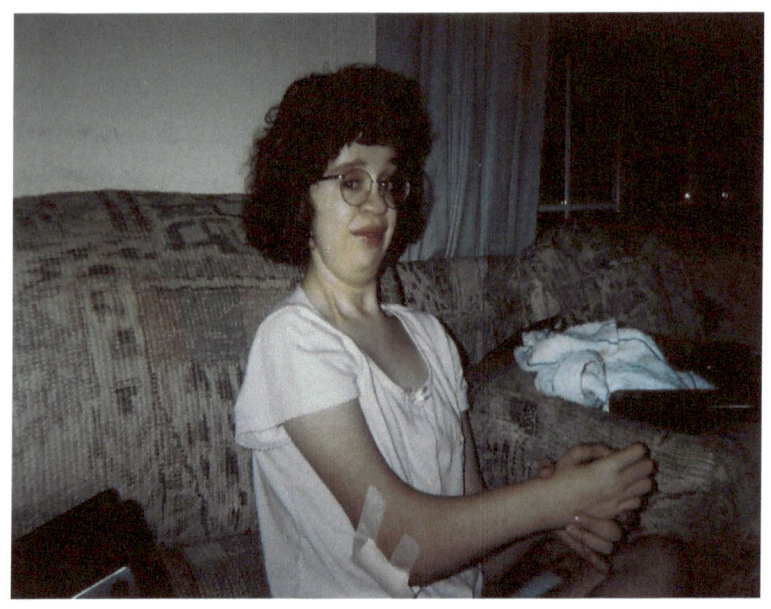

Being released from the hospital meant my determination was now the decisive factor in my arm's mobility. It was time to devise a strategic plan to defeat scar tissue, my archenemy, in a must-win situation. I decided to be on the CPM machine for two hours at a time with an hour between the splints and therapy respectively. As my mind focused on my goal, I was desperate to defeat my rival. Unfortunately, after months of agonizing pain, it appeared scar tissue was winning the battle because my arm was once again locking up. I also developed an infection from the incision location. However, that didn't mean I stopped striving for liberty.

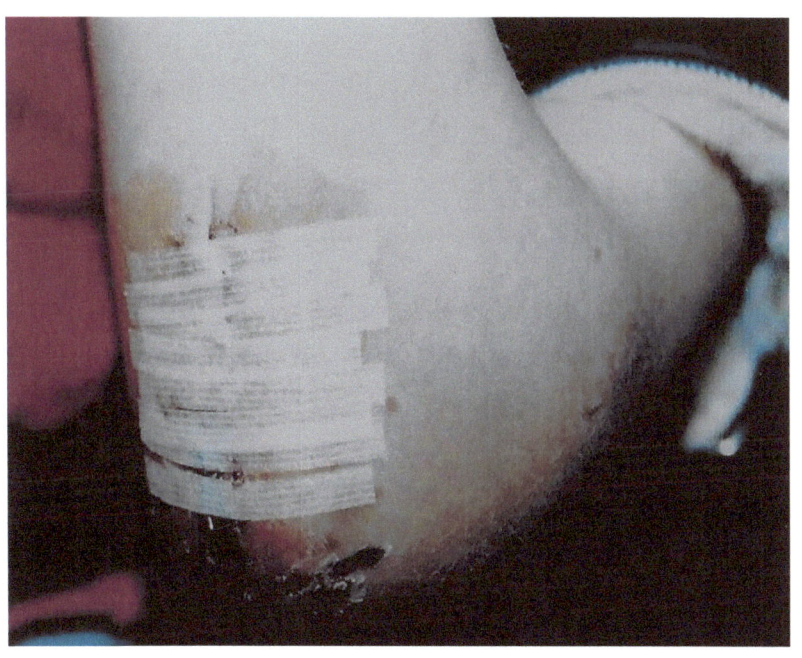

Telling Dr. Morey the unfortunate news that scar tissue won this round and an infection invaded my arm was a hard pill to swallow. Worried about Dr. Morey's reaction, it took a lot of courage to walk back into his office. I thought he took the news of the arm malfunctioning surprisingly well, considering it was my first experience with therapy after surgery. He instructed me to leave the infection alone as it would heal itself, but to use betadine ointment to speed up the process. Dr. Morey sensed my ambitious attitude. He offered to send me to Indiana University Health in Indianapolis where he thought Dr. Alexander Mih, who did his fellowship with him, could take over. Unbeknownst to him, with bewildered looks on our faces over this recommendation, we told Dr. Morey that Dr. Mih told us nothing could be done. Without hesitation, Dr. Morey said; "Oh, he can do this!" I will talk to him." It was back to square one!

Going back to a doctor who once told me there was no "magic bullet" was an intense situation. Walking back into his office was intimidating. When Dr. Mih entered the room, my mother apologized for any trouble she may have caused and explained how we found the doctor with whom he had done his fellowship. Although he seemed to remember my case, Dr. Mih didn't appear to hold a grudge over us consulting another doctor and began planning round two of elbow modification. His mission was to remove additional bone re-growth and stretch tendons. This round involved less work, but the aftermath was just another déjà vu event.

Like the first round, once Dr. Mih finished round two, I followed the same scenario. My strategy didn't change as I continued alternating between the CPM machine, splints, attending therapy three times a week, and doing home therapy. Unfortunately, as months went by, a similar pattern formed. My arm locked up once again as if there was additional bone blockage. It wasn't easy going back to a doctor who once told you nothing could be done as I feared an, 'I told you so' moment, but I refused to give up. Swallowing my pride, I walked back into his office to prove to him I wasn't quitting until my arm moved to my satisfaction.

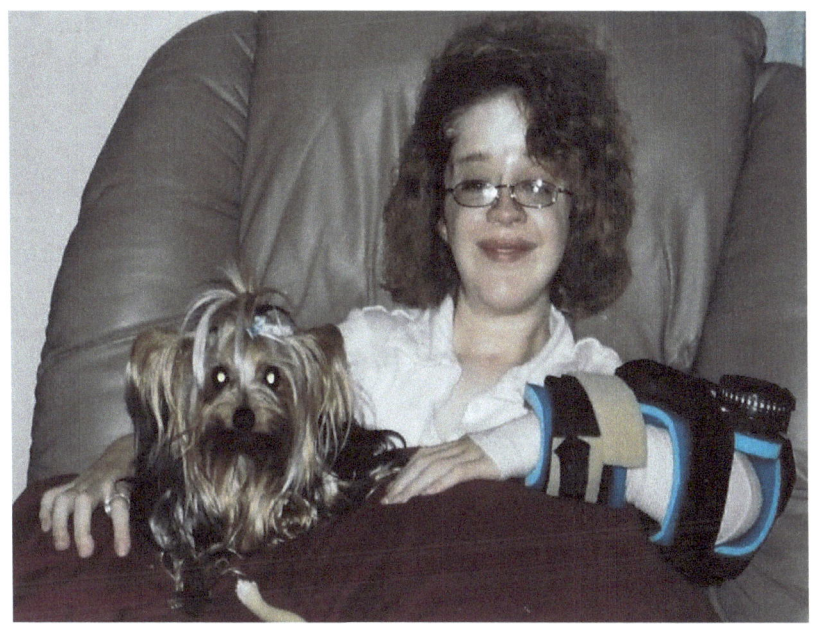

Upon entering the room, Dr. Mih evaluated my arm and thought scar tissue rather than bone re-growth caused my arm to stiffen. He instructed me to continue my plan as he thought the scar tissue had to eventually give. As told, I stuck with the same routine of flexing and extending my arm a bit longer. My arm, however, had no intentions of budging any further. Therefore, I made my presence felt, once again, at the doctor's office in order to encourage round three to achieve more mobility.

Going back and forth to the doctor to seek functional arms was getting old, but I wasn't accepting anything less. I'm sure when Dr. Mih entered the room he was thinking I had overstayed my welcome, but he wasn't willing to give up if I wasn't. We were in this together to find the answer to success. His duty was to remove more scar tissue. Scar tissue may have won the battle, but I intended to win the war.

Comparing the intensity from the first two surgeries to the third surgery was impossible. The stakes couldn't have been any higher in the third round. I knew this could be my last opportunity towards independence. If I couldn't get it moving, I would have to consider "throwing in the towel." Now, more than ever, I was aiming for liberty from my arm. It was "do or die" time. As I was being prepped for surgery, I wondered what changes I needed to make, if any, to make this sequence of surgeries a success. Rather than alter my therapy sessions, I concluded more aggressive therapy was the answer to receiving mobility. I headed into the operating room with every intention of this being my last attempt with the right arm. The anticipation of waking up from surgery was off the charts as I was eager to go to work once again in order to make my dream come true.

"Third time's the charm," occasionally holds true. This time, following repetitive surgeries and physical therapies, I was victorious because minimal scar tissues, which developed in this round, allowed my arm to miraculously move with no sign of locking up. I guess sometimes it really does take practice to make perfect. Finally, I could go back to Dr. Mih with my head held high and declare I had conquered my rival. It was nice not to have the urge to crawl under a rock because of embarrassment. My confidence strengthened enough that I later had the left arm done. Dr. Mih's mission with the left arm was the same as with the right. The aftermath treatment, on my end, concerning the CPM machine, splints, and therapy was the same grueling scenario with lots of blood, sweat, and tears. It still took three tries on the left arm, but the final try required no incision as I was put under anesthesia only to break up any scar tissue that had formed by forcing my arm to flexion and extension. Nobody really caused the first two rounds on both arms to fail because, as Thomas Edison said when explaining his light bulb, "It was "a 'thousand' step process."

Frustration from daily routines slowly diminished. While it took time, I'm now able to wash and style my hair without Mom's help. It's nice not to have to ask someone to cut up my food since I am able to hold my silverware properly. My arm now bends certain ways that makes it smoother to put clothes on. Buttoning-up shirts is less troublesome since my arm is able to reach further. Not having to ask my parents to help dress me is nice. My negative self-esteem is deteriorating since I'm able to wear make-up and put on necklaces whenever I choose. Worrying about people asking me if I have a rash has stopped because I'm able to smack mosquitos and bugs before they bite. Along with accomplishing daily routines, I was also finally able to get my driver's license. The day I realized I was no longer imprisoned in my own body was my independence day.

There is always an underlying message to a story. People who are considering having a similar operation should never let fear stop them from achieving freedom. Personal determination and willingness to work hard, however, is the key to a successful outcome. If a person is not motivated to do therapy after surgery then I don't suggest going through with the operation. Just like knee replacements, patients can't wake up from elbow surgery and expect Mother Nature to take over the healing process. As long as patients are persistent with therapy to remove scar tissue, they will be able to declare themselves victorious and independent.

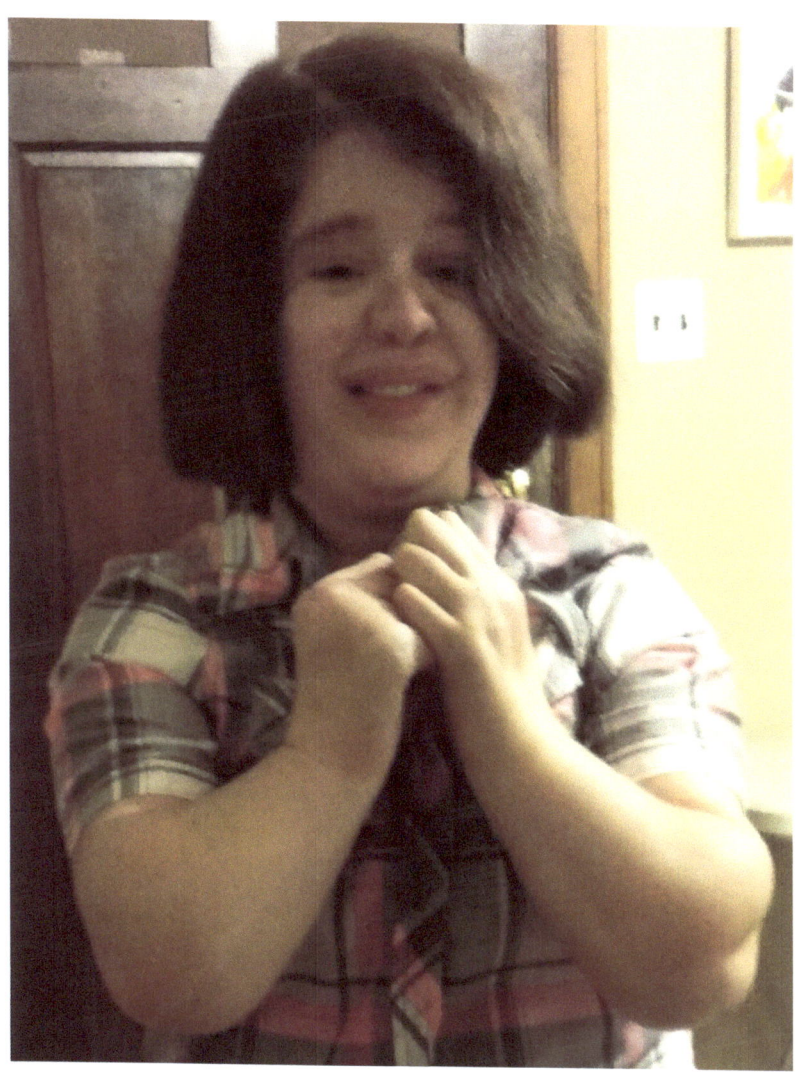

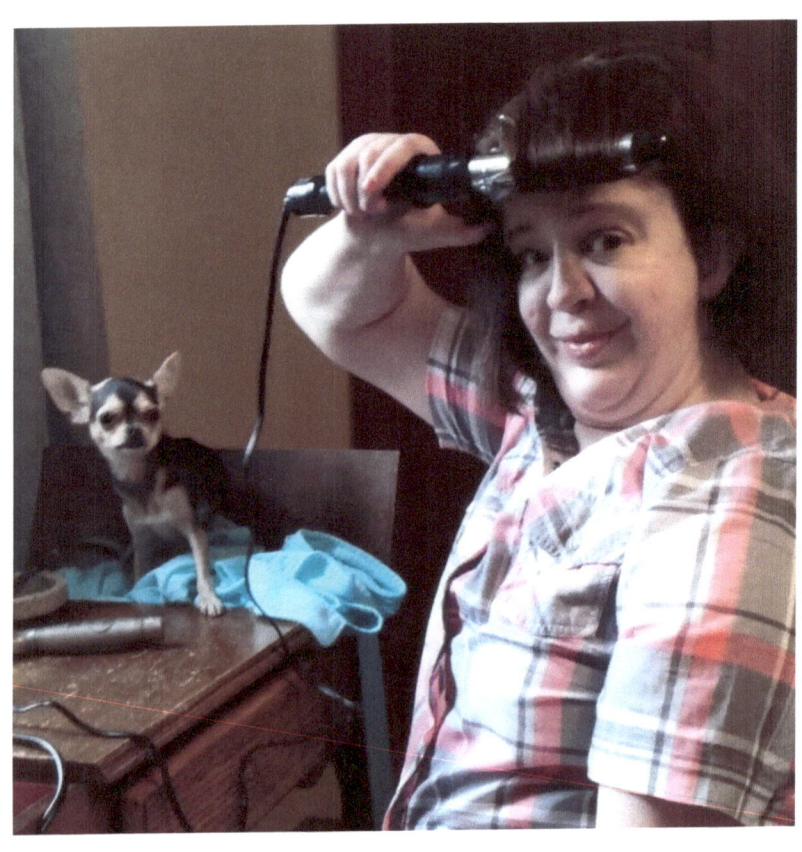

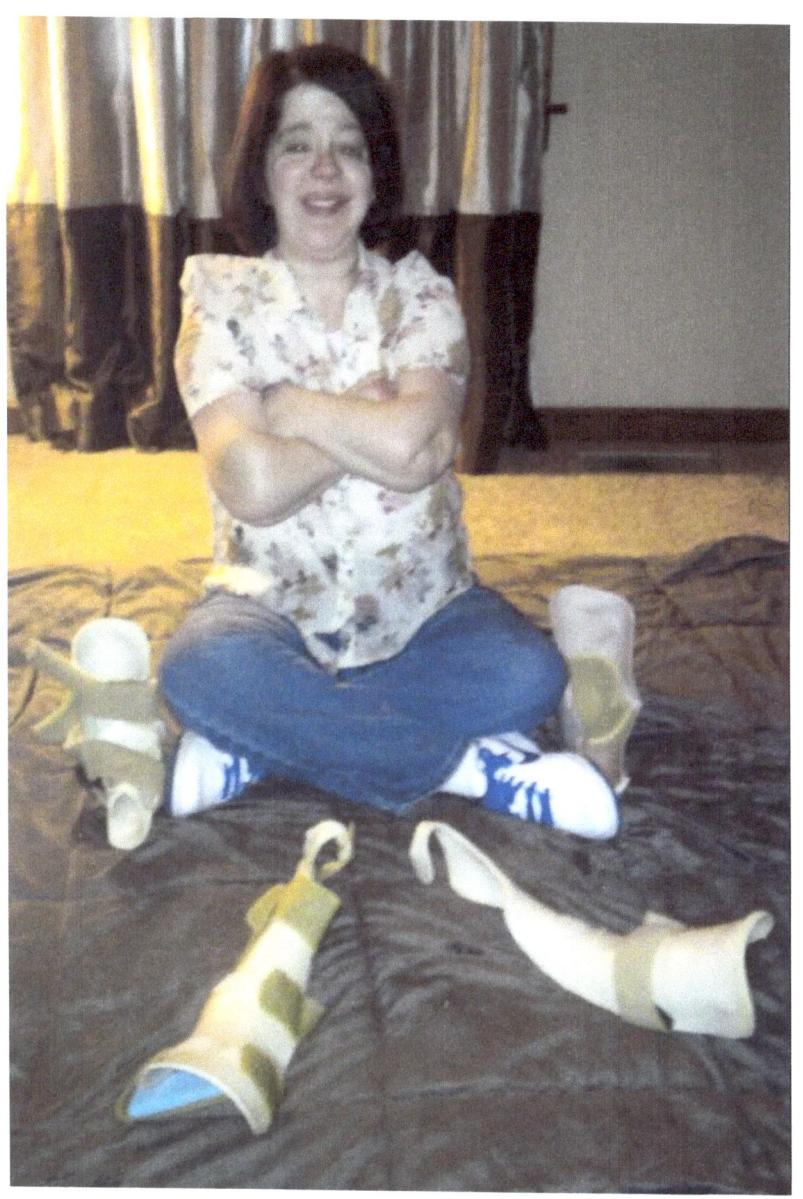

Acknowledgements

I would like to thank my parents for never giving up on me and finding a doctor who would release my elbows to give me freedom. Also, I can't thank them enough for encouraging me to reach that freedom through physical therapy. Along with my parents, I would like to thank two orthopedic doctors for having the hope of that freedom become a reality. Dr. James Morey, from Mayo Clinic, should receive credit for jump-starting my road to freedom while Dr. Alexander Mih deserves credit for me reaching it. Thank you, Dr. Morey and Dr. Mih, for not giving up on this strong-willed woman!